Syndrome

Noted details on all you need to know about syndron management

Dr Joe smith

Contents

chapter1

introduction to chronic fatique syndron

all you need to know about syndron management syndronChronic Fatigue Syndrome (CFS), also known as myalgic encephalomyelitis (ME), is a complex and debilitating disorder that affects millions of people worldwide. It is a chronic condition that causes extreme fatigue, limiting a person's ability to perform daily tasks, and can significantly impact their overall quality of life. CFS is a relatively recent discovery, and its controversies, elusive cause, and lack of definitive diagnosis and treatment have made it a challenging and misunderstood condition. The history of CFS dates back to the late 19th century, with sporadic reports of outbreaks of "chronic fatigue" in the medical literature. However, it was not until the 1930s that CFS gained more recognition when an outbreak of the illness occurred at a hospital in Los Angeles, which was later known as the "Royal Free outbreak." This outbreak involved more than 292 cases of fatigue that persisted for several weeks, accompanied by other symptoms, such as fever and abdominal pain. The hospital's medical staff initially thought this outbreak was caused by influenza, but the symptoms were not consistent with the flu. The outbreak was the first recorded incident of a post-infectious illness that would later become known as CFS. In the 1980s, there were a series of outbreaks of CFS-like symptoms that gained significant media attention and increased recognition worldwide. These outbreaks opened doors for further research into the condition, leading to the introduction of various diagnostic criteria and a better understanding of the disease. However, it wasn't until 1988, when the first official diagnostic criteria for CFS were published by the Centers for Disease Control and Prevention (CDC), that the term "Chronic Fatigue Syndrome" was officially adopted. Today, CFS is recognized as a complex and long-term condition that is characterized by severe and persistent fatigue that is not relieved by rest and is not caused by other medical conditions. According to a report by the Institute of Medicine (now known as the National Academy of Medicine), CFS affects an estimated 2.5 million people in the United States alone, with prevalence rates varying between 0.1% and 2.6% worldwide. The primary symptom of CFS is fatigue, but it is not your typical tiredness. It is a debilitating exhaustion that is not relieved by sleep, significantly impacting a person's ability to function and perform daily tasks. This fatigue is often described as a feeling of extreme exhaustion or flu-like malaise that can last for months or even years. Accompanying this fatigue are other symptoms that can include muscle and joint pain, cognitive difficulties such as brain fog and problems with concentration and memory, headaches, sore throat, enlarged lymph nodes, and unrefreshing sleep. CFS is a challenging condition to diagnose, and it can take months or even years for a proper diagnosis to be made. This is partly due to the vagueness of the symptoms and the lack of a definitive diagnostic test. Before diagnosing someone with CFS, other medical conditions that can cause similar symptoms must first be ruled out. This process can involve various tests, such as blood tests, imaging scans, and doctor consultations. Another factor contributing to the difficulty in diagnosing CFS is the lack of understanding of its underlying cause. While the exact cause of CFS is still unknown, it is believed to be a multifactorial condition that can be triggered by various factors. These include viral infections, such as Epstein-Barr virus and human herpesvirus 6, hormonal imbalances, immune dysfunction, and psychological stressors. Some experts believe that a combination of these factors may be responsible for the development of CFS. The lack of a clear understanding of the cause of CFS has also led to controversies and stigmatization of those suffering from the condition. In the past, there have been misconceptions that CFS was a psychiatric disorder or a made-up illness. This has led to the marginalization of patients and a delay in proper diagnosis and treatment. However, with more research and understanding of the condition, the attitude towards CFS has shifted, and it is now seen as a legitimate medical condition. Currently, there is no cure for CFS, but there are various management strategies that can help alleviate symptoms and improve a person's quality of life. These include a combination of pharmacological and non-pharmacological approaches such as exercise therapy, cognitive behavioral therapy, and lifestyle modifications. Medications may be prescribed to treat specific symptoms, such as pain, sleep disturbance, and depression.

The Impact of Chronic Fatigue Syndrome on Daily Life

The impact of CFS on daily life is immense, as it affects individuals physically, mentally, and emotionally, making even the simplest tasks challenging to accomplish. One of the most significant impacts of CFS on daily life is the profound and persistent fatigue experienced by individuals. Unlike tiredness caused by physical exertion, CFS fatigue is not relieved by rest or sleep, and it can be debilitating. This extreme exhaustion makes it difficult for individuals to carry out daily activities such as work, household chores, and social engagements. It can also interfere with the ability to engage in physical activities, leading to a sedentary lifestyle and further exacerbating the symptoms of CFS. The unpredictability of CFS symptoms also has a significant impact on daily life.

Individuals with CFS experience fluctuating symptoms, and what may be manageable one day can be unbearable the next. This makes it challenging to plan and organize daily tasks, as individuals may not know how much energy they will have on any given day. It can also make it challenging to maintain a regular routine, as individuals may have to constantly adjust their activities based on their current level of fatigue. Cognitive impairment, also known as "brain fog," is another common symptom of CFS that affects daily life. Individuals with CFS may experience difficulties with memory, concentration, and processing information, making it challenging to carry out tasks that require mental energy and focus. This can interfere with work, social interactions, and even simple tasks like reading and watching TV. It can significantly impact an individual's ability to think clearly and function effectively, which can lead to frustration and a sense of isolation. Apart from physical and cognitive symptoms, CFS also takes an emotional toll on individuals. The constant fatigue, pain, and other symptoms can lead to feelings of hopelessness, sadness, and anxiety. The inability to carry out daily activities and participate in social events can also lead to feelings of isolation and loneliness. This can have a significant impact on an individual's mental health and overall quality of life. Depression and anxiety are commonly associated with CFS, and addressing the emotional impact of the condition is essential for managing the condition effectively. The impact of CFS on daily life also extends to the individuals' personal relationships and social life. Due to fatigue and other symptoms, individuals with CFS may not be able to maintain a social life or participate in family activities. This can lead to strained relationships and a sense of isolation from loved ones. Moreover, the lack of understanding and awareness about CFS in the general population can lead to stigmatization, making it challenging for individuals to seek support and understanding from others. The financial impact of CFS on daily life cannot be overlooked either. The condition can affect an individual's ability to work, or even lead to prolonged periods of unemployment. This can result in financial strain and cause individuals to rely on support from family or government benefits, further adding to the emotional burden caused by the condition. The diagnosis and treatment of CFS are still evolving, and many individuals may have to try various treatments and lifestyle adjustments before finding what works for them. This can be a frustrating and overwhelming process, adding to the impact on daily life. The lack of a definitive cure for CFS also means that individuals may have to learn to manage their symptoms and adapt to a new way of living to cope with the condition long-term.

Chapter2

. Current Treatments and Management Options for Chronic Fatigue Syndrome

1. Lifestyle Changes One of the first steps in managing CFS is making lifestyle changes to help alleviate symptoms and improve overall health. This includes maintaining a balanced and healthy diet, getting enough sleep and rest, and avoiding activities and situations that can trigger or worsen symptoms. It is also important to establish a daily routine and pace daily activities to avoid overexertion. Meditation, relaxation techniques, and stress management strategies can also be beneficial in managing CFS. These techniques can help reduce stress,

improve sleep, and promote a sense of calm and well-being. Additionally, engaging in gentle forms of exercise, such as yoga, tai chi, or walking, can help improve overall physical strength and energy levels. 2. Medications Medications are often prescribed to help alleviate some of the symptoms of CFS. These may include pain relievers for muscle and joint pain, antidepressants for sleep disturbances and mood management, and medications to treat other associated conditions, such as migraines or irritable bowel syndrome. It is important to work closely with a healthcare provider to monitor the effectiveness and potential side effects of these medications. 3. Cognitive Behavioral Therapy (CBT) CBT is a type of psychotherapy that has shown promising results in managing CFS symptoms. This therapy focuses on changing unhelpful thoughts and behaviors that can contribute to anxiety, depression, and fatigue. It can also help individuals develop coping strategies for managing symptoms and improving overall function. 4. Graded Exercise Therapy (GET) GET is a structured exercise program that is designed to help individuals with CFS gradually increase their physical activity levels. This can help improve physical function and reduce fatigue without exacerbating symptoms. The goal of GET is to increase activity levels without causing a relapse, so it is important to work with a healthcare provider to develop an appropriate exercise plan. 5. Restorative Therapies A variety of restorative therapies, such as massage, acupuncture, and hydrotherapy, have been found to be helpful in managing CFS symptoms. These therapies can help reduce stress, improve sleep, and alleviate pain and muscle tension. 6. Immunomodulatory Therapy Immunomodulatory therapy involves the use of medications that modify the functioning of the immune system. This type of therapy has shown promise in treating CFS, as some studies have found evidence of immune system dysfunction in individuals with the condition. Examples of immunomodulatory medications used in CFS treatment include low-dose naltrexone and rituximab. 7. Supplements There is some evidence that certain supplements, such as vitamin B12, magnesium, and coenzyme Q10, can help alleviate symptoms of CFS. However, it is important to consult with a healthcare provider before beginning any supplementation, as these may interact with other medications or have potential side effects. 8. Pacing and Energy Management Since CFS is characterized by extreme fatigue, it is important for individuals to learn how to manage their energy levels and pace activities accordingly. This involves setting realistic goals, taking breaks when needed, and prioritizing tasks. By carefully managing energy levels, individuals can prevent overexertion and conserve energy for essential tasks. 9. Support Groups Living with CFS can be isolating and challenging, and it is important for individuals to have a support system. Joining a support group can provide a sense of community and understanding, as well as practical tips for managing symptoms and living with the condition. 10. Alternative Therapies There are a variety of alternative therapies that may be helpful in managing CFS symptoms, such as herbal remedies, homeopathy, and biofeedback. While there is limited scientific evidence to support the effectiveness of these therapies, some individuals may find relief and benefit from them.

debunking myths and misconceptions

vChapter3

About chronic fatique syndrome

Myth #1: CFS is just feeling tired all the time One of the most common and damaging misconceptions about CFS is that it is simply a case of feeling tired all the time. In reality, CFS is a multi-systemic disorder that affects not only energy levels but also cognitive function, immune system, and other bodily systems. The fatigue experienced by people with CFS is not just regular tiredness that can be relieved by a good night's sleep. It is a persistent, overwhelming exhaustion that significantly interferes with daily functioning and can last for weeks, months, or even years. Myth #2: CFS is a psychological condition Another pervasive myth about CFS is that it is a psychological condition or purely psychosomatic. This misconception can be incredibly hurtful to individuals with CFS, as it implies that their illness is not real. CFS is a medically recognized and complex condition that has been extensively researched, and there is no evidence to suggest that it is caused by psychological factors. While stress and mental health issues may contribute to the severity and management of CFS, they do not cause the condition. Myth #3: Only lazy people get CFS Another harmful misconception about CFS is that it only affects lazy and unmotivated people. This harmful stereotype not only perpetuates stigma but also undermines the severity and complexity of the condition. The reality is that CFS can affect anyone, regardless of their lifestyle or work ethic. In fact, many people with CFS were highly active and driven individuals before the onset of the illness. Myth #4: CFS is a fake illness Due to the lack of a known cause and definitive diagnostic test for CFS, some people believe that it is not a real illness. This harmful myth has been perpetuated by the media and fueled by the lack of understanding and awareness of the condition. However, CFS is a legitimate and debilitating condition that has been recognized by numerous health organizations, including the World Health Organization and the Centers for Disease Control and Prevention. Myth #5: There is a cure for CFS There is currently no known cure for CFS. While there are treatments that can help manage symptoms and improve overall quality of life, they do not offer a cure. This misconception can be particularly damaging as it gives false hope to individuals with CFS and their loved ones. It also undermines the severity and complexity of the condition, making it seem like a temporary inconvenience instead of a chronic illness. Myth #6: CFS is a women's illness Another common myth about CFS is that it primarily affects women. While women are more likely to be diagnosed with CFS, it is believed that this is due to the fact that they are more likely to seek medical help for their symptoms. It is estimated that there are just as many men with CFS as women. This misconception can be harmful as it leads to a lack of research and understanding of how the illness may present differently in men. Myth #7: CFS is caused by a viral infection It is commonly believed that CFS is caused by a viral infection, particularly the Epstein-Barr virus (EBV). While some people with CFS may have had a viral infection before developing the illness, there is no evidence to suggest that CFS is directly caused by a virus. CFS is a complex condition with a multi-factorial etiology, and no single cause has been identified. Myth #8: Exercise can cure CFS Exercise can be beneficial for individuals with CFS, but it certainly cannot cure the condition. In fact, overexertion and pushing oneself too hard can exacerbate symptoms and lead to a relapse. It is essential for individuals with CFS to engage in appropriate levels of activity and rest to effectively manage their energy levels and symptoms. Myth #9: CFS is a mild condition While some people may experience mild symptoms of CFS, for many others, it is a severe and debilitating condition. It is estimated that around 25% of people with CFS are housebound or bedbound, and many are unable to work or perform daily tasks. CFS can have a profound impact on a person's life and well-being, and it should not be dismissed as a mild condition. Myth #10: CFS is not a life-threatening illness Many people believe that CFS is not a life-threatening illness, but this is not the case. While the condition itself is not typically fatal, the severe and persistent symptoms of CFS can lead to serious complications, such as cardiovascular issues, as well as an increased risk of suicide. CFS can also significantly impact a person's mental health and overall quality of life.

Myth

The end